CHOOSE WELL

CHOOSE WELL

The ABC Coping Sentence

DR CLAIRE HAYES

BEEHIVE

Published 2023 by
Beehive Books
7–8 Lower Abbey Street
Dublin 1
Ireland
info@beehivebooks.ie
www.beehivebooks.ie

Beehive Books is an imprint of Veritas Publications.

ISBN 978 1 80097 053 3

10 9 8 7 6 5 4 3 2

A catalogue record for this book is available from the British Library.

Designed by Jeannie Swan, Beehive Books
Printed in the Republic of Ireland by SPRINT-print Ltd, Dublin

Beehive Books is a member of Publishing Ireland.

Beehive books are printed on paper made from the wood pulp of managed forests. For every tree felled, at least one tree is planted, thereby renewing natural resources.

For my mother, Joy,
in memory of my father, Liam,
and for my family,
with love and thanks.

Contents

Introduction
I choose to cope

Viktor Frankl and Edith Eger are two people who deliberately chose to cope.

Dr Frankl's experiences as a survivor of the Holocaust greatly influenced his work as a psychiatrist and psychotherapist. He emphasised the power we each have to choose our own response to whatever we experience in life and he developed a form of therapy called logotherapy. His book *Man's Search for Meaning* was originally published in 1946 and continues to be an international bestseller. Frankl died in 1997 aged ninety-two but the meaning of his life lives on through his interviews, which are easily accessible on YouTube and in his writing, including *Yes to Life: In Spite of Everything*, first published in 1946 and published in English for the first time in 2020.

Dr Edith Eger was born in 1927 and continues to draw on her experiences of surviving the Holocaust to help others in her work as a clinical psychologist. Her books *The Choice: Embrace the Possible* (2017) and *The Gift: 12 Lessons to Save Your Life* (2020) powerfully show the resilience of the human spirit, even, or maybe especially, in the face of extreme adversity. Some of her TED Talks and interviews as well as her film, *I Danced for the Angel of Death – The Dr. Edith Eva Eger Story*, are available on YouTube and will continue to help people for generations to come.

People throughout the world choose to cope with the aftermaths of the particular trauma they experience. Our daily news highlights the sufferings of people of all ages and backgrounds. War and its horrors continue to adversely affect the lives of millions. The impact of earthquakes, hurricanes, tsunamis and other so-called 'natural disasters' are exacerbated by climate change and human error. Guns are too available in many parts of the world and mass shootings are unfortunately common. Despite awareness campaigns, abuse, in all its forms, is prevalent in families and communities, tearing lives apart.

While many of us are safe from the horrors of concentration camps, war and 'natural disasters', we are not immune to life's challenges. Pressures such as disability, unemployment, illness, financial stressors and the death of people we love, collide with daily inconveniences such as traffic jams, time pressures and other people's unmet expectations.

Add to all this the trauma to which we too often subject ourselves. Taunting ourselves because we think that we are not good enough. Believing that we are not good enough and never will be. Doing things that make us feel better for a moment but which only contribute to us feeling worse in the longer term. It is not surprising that so many people experience anxiety, depression and/or addiction.

'Love your neighbour as yourself' is the core of all the world's major religions. It seems a simple enough suggestion. Yet the levels of distress in the world right now indicate that we are good neither at loving our neighbours nor ourselves. Maybe there is confusion about what it means to love ourselves. Growing up, many of us heard the phrase 'self-praise is no praise'. We witnessed parents and grandparents ensuring that everyone else had sufficient food before serving out the tiny portion that was left for themselves. Prioritising the 'self' was seen as selfish.

My work as a clinical psychologist involves people being open with me about what is really going on for them. The extent to which many of us cruelly judge, condemn and torture ourselves is shocking and disturbing. How can we stop this pattern of cruelly attacking ourselves? Few mothers give birth hoping that their babies will grow up hating themselves, comparing themselves unfavourably with others, and punishing themselves for their perceived failings. What kind of a society do we live in where behaviour like this is becoming the norm?

My experience shows me that too many of us are not good at loving either our neighbours or ourselves. Too many of us prioritise loving others, without really understanding what this means and what it involves. 'Loving others' can be misunderstood as rescuing, excusing, protecting, enabling, and sometimes even abusing, other people, who are often vulnerable and unaware that they deserve so much better. Why? Maybe because they do not love themselves enough and so do not recognise that what they give to others, in the name of love, is not love.

It is clear that challenges will never stop coming our way, so what do we do?

We choose to cope or we choose not to cope.

Choosing to cope does not mean that we have to know how we are going to cope. It simply sets us on that path.

We can benefit from the wisdom of other people who have learned to cope. I continue to learn to cope with my own life challenges. They are in no way comparable to those of Dr Frankl, Dr Eger, or billions of people worldwide. They are unique to me and yet, in many ways, they are universal. Just as I think I have managed to cope with one challenge, another one comes along. Sometimes several come together.

My way of coping is simple in some ways. I realise that what is causing me upset is usually not whatever it is, but my own reaction to it. My reaction is rooted in my early childhood experiences, my background, my personality and my own perceptions. I am learning to be kinder to myself as I acknowledge to myself, and perhaps to someone I trust, how I am feeling. Most of the time, I am honest with myself: if I feel upset, I acknowledge that I feel upset. If I feel hurt, I acknowledge that I feel hurt. If I feel scared, I acknowledge that I feel scared. This has become the first part of what I call 'The ABC Coping Sentence'.

Then I link how I feel to the reason why I feel how I feel. That is the 'B' part of the ABC Coping Sentence: 'because'. Sometimes I feel how I feel because something has happened to cause me to feel that way. Sometimes I feel how I feel because of my own thoughts and beliefs.

The 'C' part of the ABC Coping Sentence is 'choose', which is the focus of this book. For many years, the words 'but I choose to cope' inspired me to focus on how I could cope.

The ABC Coping Sentence is the last step in a three-step system I have developed to explain the key principles of cognitive behavioural therapy (CBT). CBT was developed by the American psychiatrist Aaraon Beck, building on the work of others, including the Austrian psychotherapist Albert Adler and, I suspect, Viktor Frankl.

CBT is a way of helping people to recognise the impact that their thoughts, beliefs and actions have on their feelings. I have always liked it as a way of working. I like its simplicity and its ability to empower people to make changes that turn their lives around.

You might be familiar with the Coping Triangle, which is a three-step process I have developed to explain the key principles of CBT. The first step in the process is to become aware of our thoughts, feelings and actions in relation to whatever is causing us distress and to write these on an inverted triangle.

The second step is to ask the following four questions:

- Do my feelings make sense?
- Are my thoughts 'helpful' or 'unhelpful'?
- What do I believe?
- Are my actions 'helpful' or 'unhelpful'?

The ABC Coping Sentence, the third step in using the Coping Triangle, is the focus of this book.

The ABC Coping Sentence is a process by which we can first acknowledge that our feelings make sense, based on what is happening in our lives and/or what we are thinking. In some instances, the words 'I think' are not appropriate, which is why I place them in brackets. We can easily recognise how the phrase 'I feel pain because I caught my finger in the door' makes more sense than 'I feel pain because I think I caught my finger in the door'!

However, our thoughts can cause us to feel distress even if they are not true. Picture yourself walking into a room of strangers chatting. You stand waiting for someone to include you. If asked how you were feeling in the few moments it takes for someone to acknowledge your presence, you might say, 'I feel hurt/uncomfortable/ embarrassed because they are ignoring me' or 'I feel hurt/ uncomfortable/embarrassed because I think they are ignoring me.' While it might or might not be true that you are being deliberately ignored, your feelings of hurt, discomfort and/or embarrassment make complete sense based on your own thoughts.

Do you see a difference between 'I feel upset because I am being treated unfairly' and 'I feel upset because I think I am being treated unfairly'?

Or between 'I feel angry because everything is always left up to me to do' and 'I feel angry because I think everything is always left up to me to do'?

While the reality could well be that we are being ignored, treated unfairly and left to do everything, it is our thoughts that trigger us to feel hurt, upset and angry. Our thoughts are clues to the meaning we give to certain events. The meaning itself is typically rooted in our core beliefs, which may have developed when we were very young. When someone genuinely believes what they believe, attempting to convince them that they are wrong can backfire. Such attempts can be used as further proof that the belief is accurate as people will distort whatever they see, or are told, in order to fit with their core beliefs. Most, if not all, of us do this.

The ABC Coping Sentence provides us with a different way of challenging our beliefs. Instead of wasting energy trying to challenge those beliefs, it focuses on what helpful actions we can choose to take, irrespective of what we believe and whether these beliefs are true. The ABC Coping Sentence is a tool we can use to acknowledge feelings such as hurt, upset, anger and fear, to see these as making sense based on our thoughts and/or what is happening in our world, and to focus specifically on helpful actions we can choose to take in response. Some examples are:

- 'I feel hurt because I think they are ignoring me, but I choose to give them a chance.'
- 'I feel upset because I think I am being treated unfairly, but I choose to find out if this is the case.'
- 'I feel angry because I think everything is always left up to me to do, but I choose to manage my feelings of anger responsibly.'

I am privileged to work with people of all ages and with all types of challenges. In my work with them, as well as in continuing to take care of myself as best I can, the original 'I choose to cope' has evolved to focus on *how* to cope. Some examples include 'but I choose to breathe slowly'; 'but I choose to ask for, accept and use support'; 'but I choose to be kind to myself'; and 'but I choose to remember that I am more than all of this'. I have called the endings to the ABC Coping Sentence 'Choose Well Statements'. I now know that there are an infinite number of these and the challenge in writing this book was to use the ones I personally find most useful and to share them with you in the hope that you will find some of them useful in helping you to cope.

You may like some Choose Well Statements more than others. I hope that two or three will resonate strongly enough with you for you to use them often throughout your day. My suggestion is that you read the book in whatever way you choose. That might mean starting at the beginning and going to the end. It might mean looking at the Table of Contents and seeing if there is a particular Choose Well Statement that you are drawn to, or it might mean opening the book at random.

I have come to appreciate the power we each have to choose to make our lives easier. We cannot stop challenges arising. We cannot prevent a global pandemic, severe hurricanes, or droughts. We cannot ensure that the people we love will live forever. We cannot live our lives free from pain, upset, disappointment, fear or anger – nor might we want to, as these experiences enrich our lives in ways that we might appreciate only years later.

We can, however, choose how we respond to whatever causes us pain. Sometimes, it might seem as if we have no choice about feeling upset. But we do. We always do. We can choose to respond to life's challenges in ways that make us more resilient. We can choose to be honest with ourselves about the impact a particular experience has on us. We can choose to ask for help. We can choose to accept help. We can choose to learn from everything that happens to us. We can choose to use our most difficult and challenging experiences to help others. We can choose to make our lives count.

I hope that you will enjoy discovering Choose Well Statements that resonate with you.

I feel … because I (think) … but I choose to:

Cope

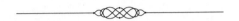

For many years, 'I choose to cope' was my only suggestion for how to end the ABC Coping Sentence.

Regardless of whatever happens to us in life, we have a choice: to cope or not to cope.

Choosing to cope may not be easy.

It can be hard to raise our hands and ask for support to help us cope.

It can be even harder to accept it.

Choosing to cope may involve us experiencing deep distress as we turn to face our challenges.

I feel … because I (think) … but I choose to:

Breathe slowly

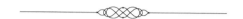

The miracle of life means that we breathe without thinking about it.

Sometimes it can be hard to breathe.

We might catch our breath, hold our breath, or even breathe so quickly that we hyperventilate.

I suggest linking the words 'I choose to breathe slowly' with this effective breathing exercise:

- Tighten your non-dominant hand while breathing in, thinking, 'I choose to breathe slowly.'
- Hold your breath for three seconds and breathe out while relaxing your hand.
- Repeat this in cycles of threes, several times throughout the day.

Notice how simply thinking, 'I choose to breathe slowly' can help your breathing to slow down and allow you to become a little more relaxed.

I feel … because I (think) … but I choose to:

Consider that maybe I'm okay

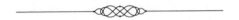

Maybe I am okay.

This is very effective for those moments when we really don't think we are okay.

One example might be, 'I feel upset because I think that I am not good enough – but maybe I'm okay.'

'Maybe' is a very powerful word.

Try it and see how often you can use these words in a week!

I feel … because I (think) … but I choose to:

Consider that maybe it's okay

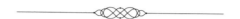

The short version of 'I choose to consider that maybe I'm okay' is 'Maybe it's okay.'

We tend to scare and torture ourselves by picturing dire consequences for what we have done and what we haven't done.

We worry about how we are going to cope in the future if our worst fears come true, whatever they may be.

Reassurance from others tends not to be effective as no one can guarantee that our worst fears, however unlikely, will not come true.

The key is considering that, even if our worst fears do come true, maybe it's still okay.

Maybe once the 'worst' has happened, we will be able to relax and see things from a different perspective.

Maybe we will get help from people we would never expect to help us.

Maybe it really is okay.

I feel … because I (think) … but I choose to:

Learn from this

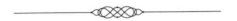

Many years ago, I was behind an elderly lady in a queue. I was in a hurry and was dismayed to see her slowly rummage in her pockets and purse for small change to pay for her purchases.

I could feel myself becoming more and more impatient.

I know that the lady and the young girl serving her were aware of my sighs of frustration.

To my horror, I began to tap my foot with impatience and noticed both of them glancing nervously at me. When I got back to my car, I viciously berated myself for how I had behaved.

As I was heading to work, I knew that I did not have the luxury of beating myself up for the rest of the day, so I decided to use the ABC Coping Sentence to help restore my sense of balance.

'I feel embarrassed and ashamed because of how I behaved just now but …'

It took me a little while to get the perfect end to this sentence but, when I did, I knew it was exactly right:

'… I choose to learn from this.'

This has become one of my favourite and most effective Choose Well Statements. It was too late for me to go back to the elderly lady and apologise for my impatient behaviour, but I could definitely learn from it in order to manage my feelings of impatience more appropriately in the future.

I feel … because I (think) … but I choose to:

Take my power back

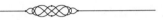

Anyone who has read or listened to my story 'The Elephant and the Mouse' in my book *Finding Hope in the Age of Anxiety* will know why 'I choose to take my power back' is one of my favourite Choose Well Statements to complete the ABC Coping Sentence.

I have seen people of all ages with all sorts of fears courageously take their power back by deliberately doing the opposite of what they think will make them feel better.

This often results in them actually feeling worse in the short term.

However, the long-term benefits are enormous.

I know many people who are now able to travel by air, use lifts, walk up an escalator, speak in groups, attend school, college or work, or even say 'No' to excessive demands.

They each successfully took their power back from fears such as feeling anxious, from the idea of making a spectacle of themselves or of letting someone down.

For most of them, taking their power back was not easy, but it was definitely liberating.

I feel … because I (think) … but I choose to:

Keep taking my power back

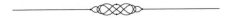

Taking our power back can be a wonderful experience.

It can also be incredibly difficult.

Just as chemotherapy often makes people who have cancer feel worse, taking our power back from our fear can initially increase our levels of anxiety.

This is why it is essential that we keep doing it, even if we feel anxious and even if we think that we are not making any progress.

It is only by choosing to keep taking our power back that our anxieties reduce, and we begin to feel strong and good about ourselves.

I feel … because I (think) … but I choose to:

Recognise the pattern

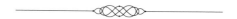

We all have patterns.

Some patterns are healthy, such as brushing our teeth twice a day.

Some patterns make other people's lives easier, such as cleaning up after ourselves when we make a mess.

Some patterns can be very destructive.

These include:

- Criticising ourselves and others for not being 'good enough'

- Relying on alcohol, sugar and/or other substances to feel better, and

- Excessively seeking reassurance.

It is also too easy to fall into a pattern of talking about what we see as 'wrong' in the world, dragging others and ourselves down.

Before we can change our destructive patterns, however, we first choose to recognise them.

I feel … because I (think) … but I choose to:

Keep changing the pattern

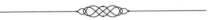

Choosing to change our destructive patterns can be liberating.

It can be even more liberating to change, and then to choose to keep changing, patterns that we no longer need.

This can be exhausting, however, and sometimes it can be tempting to fall back into old patterns.

Choosing to keep changing destructive patterns by focusing on exercising regularly, eating and sleeping well, and reflecting on whether our patterns really serve us, means that new, healthy patterns become easier and more automatic over time.

I feel … because I (think) … but I choose to:

Recognise and appreciate what is going well

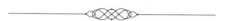

How many of us instinctively focus on what is not going well? Sometimes, it is hard to even see what *is* going well. It is as if we are 'hardwired' to notice danger, but fail to see the many things that *are* going well. And, if they are pointed out to us, we may dismiss rather than appreciate them.

I remember a child telling me once about how awful another child in his class was. He spent about ten minutes listing everything that he disliked about this boy. I listened and then asked him to tell me one good thing about the other boy. He looked at me in shock, wondering if I had heard anything he had said.

'There's nothing good about him,' he vigorously insisted.

'There has to be at least one good thing,' I responded.

After a few minutes of him repeatedly telling me that there wasn't, I asked if I could suggest one:

> 'It's good that he's not your brother and so will not be having dinner with you tonight.'

I still smile when I remember the look of absolute horror that passed over the child's face at the mere thought of being related to the boy he disliked so much. This was followed a moment later by a look of complete relief.

He had recognised that I was right. The boy he disliked was not his brother – a fact he definitely appreciated!

I feel … because I (think) … but I choose to:

Remind myself that when I am a lot older this won't matter

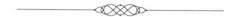

Some concerns can consume us.

Reminding ourselves that they will not matter when we are a lot older can give us a sense of perspective.

This sentence is not universally applicable as there are some things that will always matter, regardless of whatever age we reach. Poor health or sad news about someone we love are two examples.

However, reminding ourselves that some concerns are time-limited can be very powerful for helping us cope with a range of issues that cause us great distress when they occur.

Some examples include moments when someone does something that upsets us, such as accidentally breaking a precious vase.

Other examples include moments when someone seems to deliberately treat us badly; for example, damaging our car in a car park and driving away without leaving contact details.

Deliberately thinking, 'I feel angry and upset because I think that person was unfair, but I choose to remind myself that this won't matter when I am older' can be very liberating.

I feel … because I (think) … but I choose to:

Let it go

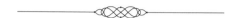

Few people live without experiencing moments of upset, distress, regret or hurt. Such moments can be difficult to experience at the time. They can be even more difficult years later when we are suddenly reminded of them.

What would it be like if we deliberately allowed ourselves to feel the pain of these moments – and then let it go?

Yes, this can be very difficult to do, particularly if we think that we are 'in the right'.

However, it can be freeing to really let go of something that caused us pain.

If there is something that continues to niggle and upset you weeks, months, or even years later, despite your best efforts to let it go, talk to someone you trust and get their support to help you let it go.

One powerful way of letting go is to use imagery.

Picture yourself getting into a boat. There is enough room for you, but not for all the resentments, worries and upsets that you are carrying as luggage.

On the shore beside the boat is an enormous recycling bin. See how much of this excess baggage you have been carrying that you can simply leave behind.

I feel ... because I (think) ... but I choose to:

Remember that you are more than this

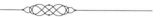

When you are feeling particularly awful, it can be uplifting to remember that you are more than this.

You are more than your feelings.

You are more than your thoughts.

You are more than your beliefs.

You are more than your actions.

You are more than your circumstances.

You are more than your stories.

Other people are more than their feelings, thoughts, beliefs, actions, circumstances and stories, too.

I feel … because I (think) … but I choose to:

Grieve my way

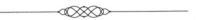

Doing things 'our way' is our right once we stay within legal limits. But there are times when it can be hard to figure out what exactly is 'our way'.

I think that this can apply to grieving. You may have heard of the five stages of grief that were first described by the Swiss-American psychiatrist Elisabeth Kübler-Ross: denial, anger, bargaining, depression and acceptance. We know that we are not 'supposed' to follow the steps from denial to acceptance but can bounce instead from one to another and back again many, many times. In the foreword of her last book, Kübler-Ross and her co-author, David Kessler, wrote that, 'There is no correct way or time to grieve.'

We know that grieving a loss is key to moving on from it, but that doesn't mean that it is easy or fast.

Grief can be intense. It can be scary. It can seem overwhelming. It can wait until we are ready for it and sometimes this may be years after we experienced the loss.

There are many books on grief. My favourite continues to be *The Courage to Grieve* by Judy Tatelbaum. While it may be tempting to advise others how to grieve, grieving is something that we each discover how to do in our own way.

I feel … because I (think) … but I choose to:

Remember the good times

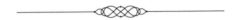

We are all familiar with the advice to 'live in the now', rather than in the past or the future.

However, it can be important, healthy and desirable to remember the good times.

I tend to do this when I am sitting in my dentist's chair – instead of focusing on the 'now', I deliberately think of special times in my life. Doing this distracts me from the noise of the drill and definitely helps me relax.

It is natural to remember good times when reminiscing with old friends and family we don't see very often.

It might not be as easy to do this when we are struggling to cope with challenges such as the death of someone we love, the breakup of a relationship, the ending of a friendship, or even retirement.

Our lives right now might seem worse by comparison, but remembering the good times can give us hope that we will have good times again in the future.

I feel … because I (think) … but I choose to:

Remember that today is today

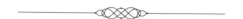

Does it seem easier to think about your past or your future than to think about today? As children, we were guided and encouraged. Think of the many hours you spent preparing for some future event. You may have studied for exams. You may have trained for an important match. You may have practised for a music competition. It is easy to live our whole lives like that, preparing for a tomorrow that we hope will somehow be easier than today.

The years fly by. They really do. We accumulate yesterdays and, as we get older, do not know how many tomorrows we might have left. Our todays can get squeezed between them.

A powerful quote by the American author Annie Dillard is: 'How we spend our days is of course how we spend our lives.'

Choosing to remember that today is today opens us up to making the very most of this precious gift we have – the present.

I feel ... because I (think) ... but I choose to:

Make this experience count

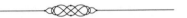

There are times in life that are difficult.

Choosing to make these experiences count can instantly empower us.

We can acknowledge how upset and distressed we feel while deliberately choosing to make our experience count.

We might not know yet *how* it can count but choosing to make it count is a great start.

We might learn a lot from the experience that we can use in time to help others.

I feel … because I (think) … but I choose to:

Let my future be my future

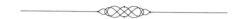

Worrying about the future is understandable. It can be unrealistic and unfair to expect someone who is struggling with poor health, relationship difficulties, financial worries and/or a host of other challenges not to worry about their future. Worrying excessively, however, can be like throwing petrol on a fire. It can also keep us paralysed, frightened and stuck.

Anticipating the future is understandable, but sometimes we miss what is happening in the present as we yearn for some future event to occur.

Do you remember being little and impatiently waiting for your birthday, or some other future event? Many of us still do this. We wait for exams to be over, for an interview to be successful; for concerts, holidays or retirement. Future events that have not happened yet can dominate our present.

When this happens, it can be powerful to acknowledge that 'I feel … because (I think) I will not be good enough, but I choose to let my future be my future.'

I feel … because I (think) … but I choose to:

Enjoy discovering how capable I actually am

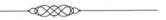

Have you noticed how young people often focus on what they cannot do rather than what they can?

This can be particularly obvious coming up to exam time.

'Studying' can become a word to describe worrying, procrastinating, distracting, eating, drinking, texting, blaming, and even paralysis.

A powerful Choose Well Statement such as: 'I feel upset because I think I have left it too late to do anything, but I choose to enjoy discovering how capable I actually am' can work wonders!

I feel ... because I (think) ... but I choose to:

Listen to myself with love, respect and gratitude

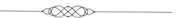

You could choose to rephrase this as 'I choose to listen to myself with love, I choose to listen to myself with respect, and I choose to listen to myself with gratitude.' I like the three words, love, respect and gratitude, used together at those times when you are treating yourself cruelly.

Let's take an example: you have a decision to make. You ask others for their opinions and listen to their responses. If they are people you love, you may listen with love as well as with respect and gratitude. But while you listen to them, you might not be listening to yourself.

What is your instinct? Is this decision the right one for you? Is this a decision that is going to impact the rest of your life? Do you have enough information right now to make this decision?

If the decision is one that keeps you awake at night, how are you responding to yourself? You may feel scared, upset or pressured. You may have thoughts such as 'I don't know what to do', 'I can't make the right decision' and 'I'm afraid of making a mistake.' You may then feel annoyed with yourself, thinking, 'What is wrong with me? Why can't I make this decision? This is ridiculous.'

It is so much kinder to acknowledge your feelings and see them as making sense in the context of the decision you need to make, as well as being a reaction to your own thoughts, and then firmly and gently choose to listen to yourself with love, respect and gratitude.

I feel … because I (think) … but I choose to:

Value what I do

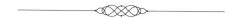

'Ah, it wasn't much, anyone could have done it' is something we may say in response to a compliment. 'It wasn't much' might have been a beautiful meal, an amazing painting or a practical task such as directing traffic at a funeral. 'Anyone could have done it' may have some truth in it, but 'anyone' didn't do it – you did it.

Why do so many of us minimise what we do? Is it that we don't want to be seen as 'big-headed'? Is it because we genuinely consider our contributions to be something that anyone else could have done?

You have your own unique fingerprints. You have your own unique style. You have your own unique way of doing things. Often, when you do something for someone else, no one else could have done it the way you did. Often, it is worth more than you realise.

I invite you to notice what you do, how you do it and, most importantly, to choose to value it.

I feel … because I (think) … but I choose to:

Forgive myself

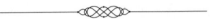

Many self-help books talk about the importance of forgiveness.

It can be much easier to forgive others than to forgive ourselves.

Every person who has ever lived has made mistakes.

We all do things that we regret. We all say things that we regret. We all wish that we could turn the clock back.

We can't do that but we can choose what to do with our regrets.

We can blame ourselves harshly. We can sentence ourselves to punishment with no parole.

Or we can choose to make amends as best we can, we can choose to learn from our mistakes, and we can choose to forgive ourselves for not being exactly how we wanted to be.

I feel … because I (think) … but I choose to:

Cherish myself

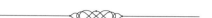

'Wait a minute,' do I hear you say?

'Self-forgiveness? Yes.

Self-love? Maybe – but self-cherishing?

That is just ridiculous!'

Why?

Why is it seen as self-indulgent, 'silly', or even wrong to cherish ourselves?

What does cherishing yourself mean to you? One definition of 'cherish' is to care and protect someone lovingly.

The word cherish sounds gentle and powerful. The action of cherishing is definitely gentle and powerful.

How can we possibly ever fully cherish others if we do not cherish ourselves?

I feel … because I (think) … but I choose to:

Enjoy myself

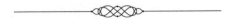

There are moments when it is so easy to enjoy myself.

There are other moments when it is not.

When I am supposed to be relaxing, I can sometimes notice my head filling with anxious thoughts.

When I catch myself wondering whether I did something well enough, or worrying about whether I will do something well enough, I notice that this distracts me from where I am, regardless of whether I am on my own or with friends.

When I notice myself having these thoughts, I deliberately tell myself that I choose to enjoy myself.

It always works.

I feel … because I (think) … but I choose to:

Accept myself

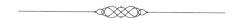

One of the ways we can cherish ourselves is to accept ourselves.

This can be extraordinarily difficult to do.

We all do things that we wish we hadn't done. Things that we would prefer other people to not know about.

Things that we probably feel ashamed of.

Accepting ourselves is accepting that we are human and that part of being human means sometimes falling short of our own standards, until we choose to do things differently.

Rejecting ourselves because of our human failings is not fair or helpful. Instead, we can choose to treat ourselves in the same way we are encouraged to treat young children when they misbehave:

'I love you – but I do not like your behaviour.'

By fully accepting ourselves, we can become better at separating ourselves from our behaviour.

What would it be like if we all decided to accept ourselves as we are, without waiting until we reached 'perfection'?

Accepting ourselves means that we stop apologising for who we are and, instead, focus on being and doing the best we can.

I feel … because I (think) … but I choose to:

Love myself

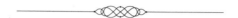

The words 'You really love yourself, don't you?' have become a terrible insult.

Seemingly, the last thing we are ever meant to do is love ourselves!

Doesn't this seem bizarre?

How can we ever love anyone else if we do not love ourselves?

Maybe the confusion is to do with what the word 'love' really means.

It is not about indulging ourselves at the expense of others.

Loving ourselves means recognising and valuing our own worth. What does 'choosing to love yourself' mean to you?

I feel … because I (think) … but I choose to:

Be kind to myself

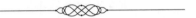

One of life's mysteries is how we can be so kind to other people and so cruel to ourselves.

I discovered the power of choosing to be kind to myself when my 'inner critic' went completely out of control.

Instead of automatically believing whatever cruel thoughts I had about myself, I deliberately focused on being kind to myself.

I began to sing 'I choose to be kind to myself' to the tune of 'Mary had a little lamb'. To my amazement, I soon noticed myself responding differently to mistakes I made or thought I had made.

Instead of berating myself savagely, the words 'I choose to be kind to myself' became my automatic response, followed by self-compassion and kindness.

I have shared this with many people and encouraged them to give themselves a gentle hand massage with beautiful hand cream, while they sing.

I am constantly amazed at how effective this simple exercise is in helping people be kinder to themselves.

The Beatles emphasised that all we need is love. We also need to be kind to ourselves as well as to others!

I feel … because I (think) … but I choose to:

Nurture myself

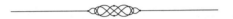

The ability to nurture ourselves may take some practice.

While it is similar to taking care of ourselves, the word 'nurture' invites us to move beyond the idea of 'taking care', to the notion of cherishing and protecting.

A valuable question to ask ourselves at particularly upsetting moments is: 'What can I choose to do to nurture myself right now?'

If this is too hard, it might be easier to think of someone who loves us and ask, 'How would that person nurture me right now?' Another option is to think of someone we love and ask, 'How would I nurture that person if they were experiencing what I am experiencing right now?'

Choosing to nurture ourselves is an important first step in doing that – more important than we might realise.

I feel … because I (think) … but I choose to:

Give myself a hug

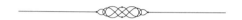

During the recent global pandemic, we were told to keep our distance from almost everyone. Handshakes and hugs became a thing of the past. A young Irish child, Alan King, captured hearts when he appeared on national television holding up his 'virtual hug' (his drawing of a heart with the words 'A hug for you'), an idea that spread and inspired people of all ages.

I missed hugs during those years more than I can describe.

At one point I remember saying to myself, 'I feel really upset because I miss hugs right now but I choose to give myself a hug.'

My 'self-hug' took a bit of practice and for a long time was a poor substitute for a hug from someone else.

As the months went by, choosing to give myself a hug took on a new meaning. It focused me on treating myself with gentleness and kindness. It only took a moment and became a practical tool for me to use whenever I felt overwhelmed, sad or lonely.

There are times when we are literally alone and there is no one to give us a hug.

Those might be the best times to choose to give ourselves one.

I feel … because I (think) … but I choose to:

Ask for support

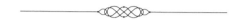

Why is asking for help so difficult?

Why do so many of us see 'asking for support' as synonymous with being weak?

I know that asking for support takes courage and is not always easy.

Thoughts such as 'I should be able to do this on my own' and 'I can't impose on other people' can make it even more difficult to ask for help.

We might assume that we are a nuisance. We might think that others see us as 'weak'. We might protect ourselves from not getting support by not asking in the first place.

Let's give other people a chance to help us when we need it.

Choose to ask for support.

I feel … because I (think) … but I choose to:

Accept support

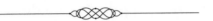

Asking for support is one thing, accepting support is another thing entirely!

We can all give support.

We can all have support offered to us.

Choosing to *accept* support can be hard if we prefer to do things on our own. Choosing to accept support can be powerful as we discover that we are not, after all, on our own.

I feel … because I (think) … but I choose to:

Remember that I have the right to say 'Yes'

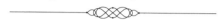

When I was nineteen years old, I spent a summer working in America as a camp counsellor. Prior to leaving Ireland, I attended a preparation course that emphasised the following three points:

(1) Americans tend to be very hospitable. (2) When they offer hospitality, it is because they want to and not because they have to. (3) If any of us wanted to accept an offer of hospitality, we needed to say 'Yes please' immediately.

We were firmly told that Americans would take us at our word if we said, 'No, thank you', and not ask twice.

The character Mrs Doyle in the television comedy *Father Ted* is known for insisting that people have a cup of tea, regardless of whether they want one or not.

There is some truth in this as, in Ireland, it is somehow considered polite to say, 'No thank you' when first offered something.

It often only seems acceptable to say, 'Yes please' when asked for the third or fourth time.

Just think how much easier life would be if we remember that we have the right to say 'Yes' when we want to!

I feel ... because I (think) ... but I choose to:

Remember that I have the right to say 'No'

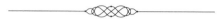

It might seem obvious that if we have the right to say 'Yes', then we also have the right to say 'No'.

Have you noticed how it can be very difficult to say 'No' even if we mean it?

Too often we say 'Yes' instead of 'No' so that we will not be seen as 'selfish', 'foolish', or simply 'awkward'.

The world would be so much clearer and more honest if we could say 'No' when we mean 'No'.

I feel ... because I (think) ... but I choose to:

Allow myself time to decide

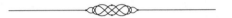

Sometimes we are under pressure to make decisions quickly.

Sometimes we simply don't have enough information to decide.

Choosing to allow ourselves time to decide can ease the pressure.

Choosing to allow ourselves time to decide can take courage.

It can lead us to saying 'No' to others who may want us to decide more quickly.

It can lead us to saying 'Yes' to what we know is truly right for us.

I feel … because I (think) … but I choose to:

Follow my instincts

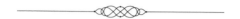

People sometimes tell me that they do not know what their instincts are. They can be so used to doing what they are told, or not doing what they are told, that they have never asked themselves what is right for them to do.

An effective exercise I have developed can help us pay attention to our instincts. Ask someone to read the following four sentences while you listen with your eyes closed. If what they say is correct, reply 'Yes' and, if it is incorrect, reply 'No'.

- 'You love where you live right now.'
- 'Your favourite food is fried banana.'
- 'Your idea of a dream holiday is a month on your own on an island off the coast of Scotland.'
- 'You find it easy to resist temptation.'

You might have been surprised by how quickly and easily you knew the correct answers. Pay particular attention to *how* you knew an answer was 'Yes' or 'No'. Some people describe 'Yes' as a physical feeling in their chest while 'No' is described with an automatic shake of the head.

We all have different ways of knowing what is right for us and, the more attentive we are to our own 'Yes' and 'No', the better we will be able to choose to follow our instincts.

I feel … because I (think) … but I choose to:

Question my beliefs

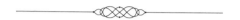

The process of identifying and challenging core beliefs is the focus of much of my work. Many of us are driven by underlying core beliefs, which, over time, can become dangerous. Beliefs such as 'I am not good enough', 'No one will understand', 'People will always let you down', 'I can't' and 'It doesn't matter' can lead us to experience life as being more difficult than it has to be.

Simply choosing to question our beliefs opens our minds to other possibilities. Maybe someone will understand. Maybe people are inherently good. Maybe what we do does matter.

When I was a teenager, I met someone from a completely different background to me. He was Jewish American and I was Catholic Irish. He explained that while he thought Jesus Christ had been a very good man, he was not the Messiah; the Messiah was going to come into the world and this could happen any day. I remember saying, 'Well, if what you believe is right, then what I believe is wrong, and if what I believe is right, then what you believe is wrong.'

For the first time, I asked myself what I believed and whether I really believed it.

About twenty-five years later, I had a similar experience in a Buddhist monastery. As I listened to the teachings of the Buddha, I was struck by many similarities to what I thought Jesus had taught. One beautiful Buddhist nun told me that the Dalai Lama encouraged people to deepen their own faith as opposed to converting to Buddhism or another religion. It was time once again for me to question what I believed and whether I really believed it.

I believe in human goodness. I believe in the power of the human spirit. I believe that everyone is free to believe or not to believe in something bigger than each of us. Ultimately, I believe in the wisdom at the core of every major religion: 'Love your neighbour as yourself.'

What do you believe?

I feel … because I (think) … but I choose to:

Do what is right for me

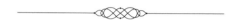

People can be very supportive. They want us to be well and they want us to do well. They might suggest, advise, recommend, and even tell us what they think we *should* do. It is tempting to do exactly what they say, particularly if we like pleasing them, but that may not be the right thing for us. It is also not possible to please everyone as we typically get conflicting suggestions, advice and recommendations.

People who like a particular car will recommend it. People who don't like a particular place to visit will advise against going there. People who have found a particular health treatment to work for them may assume that it will also work for you and may be annoyed if you don't at least try it.

Don Miguel Ruiz's book *The Four Agreements: A Practical Guide to Personal Freedom* teaches us to challenge underlying beliefs and to make the following four agreements with ourselves as well as with the world:

1. Be impeccable with your word.
2. Don't take anything personally.
3. Don't make assumptions.
4. Always do your best.

While each of these four points work well as individual Choose Well Statements in their own right, if you choose to do what is right for you, you may automatically end up doing them all.

I feel … because I (think) … but I choose to:

Pray

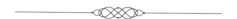

A priest friend describes prayer as 'a vital and essential communication with God that can take many forms'.

Reactions to the word 'God' can be forceful and divisive. I like the line from Max Ehrmann's poem 'Desiderata':

'Therefore, be at peace with God, whatever you conceive Him to be.'

Throughout history, people have instinctively turned to prayer to help them cope when tragedy strikes and to express gratitude for when times are good.

The Internet is often criticised but it can be a wonderful treasure trove when used responsibly. For example, Father Malachy Hanratty's book *Discoveries in Prayer* is free to download.

Googling 'how to pray' from whatever religious or spiritual perspective that works for you can lead you to some beautiful prayers and psalms that can be very helpful if you choose to pray.

I feel … because I (think) … but I choose to:

Act on my complaints

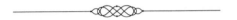

It is usually easy to notice when something is wrong. It can be harder to take powerful action to make improvements. Thoughts such as 'I don't want to be a nuisance', 'Nobody else seems to be bothered' or 'It doesn't really matter' can make it harder for us to make a complaint.

If we have complained before and nothing changed, we might also think, 'What's the point?' and feel powerless.

You may have heard the saying, 'Bad things happen when good people do nothing.' Acting on our complaints can be powerful for us and can also make a real difference to others.

Acting on our complaints means that we deal with them rather than allowing them to build up and fester. It means that we practise being assertive rather than passive or passive-aggressive.

Choosing to act on our complaints makes us consider how exactly to do that. There are times when a polite phone call is adequate; there are other times when it is important to make a formal, written complaint. We also have the choice to let go whatever we are unhappy with and not carry it with us.

The choice is ours.

I feel … because I (think) … but I choose to:

Take the initiative

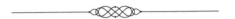

Some people enjoy being leaders. Some people are described as 'natural-born leaders'.

It can be tempting to stand back and allow others lead. That way, we protect ourselves from accusations of leading others astray. We don't have to take responsibility for the direction we choose.

Not leading means that we can never be accused of leading others astray or making the 'wrong' choice. But there can be disadvantages in holding ourselves back by not taking the initiative.

I remember once arriving on a train from Switzerland at a small town in Italy. I had only three hours before taking the train back across the border. This was before the European Union and, while I had Swiss francs, I had no Italian lire. The first place to visit when I got off the train was the local bank to change money to get a pizza and an ice cream! I was discovered there by two fellow travellers who spoke English. They were delighted to haul me outside to meet a group of people they had gathered on the train. Like me, everyone had only three hours to explore the town before going back to Switzerland.

People argued about where they should go – apparently, the clear understanding was that everyone had to go together. Some wanted to see a church while others wanted to go shopping. I watched for a few minutes before realising that my own time was ticking away. While there are many times I enjoy being with others, this was not one of them.

Food did not seem to be on anyone else's agenda so I quietly chose to take the initiative to do what I wanted, even if they thought I was rude. I did so even though I was going to miss out on whatever the group finally agreed to do. I did so and I celebrated that I did so – with a pizza and an ice cream!

I feel … because I (think) … but I choose to:

Invite others to lead

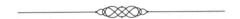

Some people find it easier to follow than to lead.

This may be due to lack of self-confidence, a preference for allowing others to lead, laziness, or many other reasons.

Supporting others to take the lead is important.

Every leader reaches the moment when someone else must take over.

History has taught us too many lessons about what happens when one person is allowed to lead, and millions stand by to watch.

We are surrounded by many amazing potential leaders.

They may not want to push themselves forward.

Think what good they can do in accepting our invitation to lead.

I feel … because I (think) … but I choose to:

Support others to make their own choices

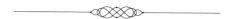

One way to manage feelings of frustration when others appear to dither is to remind ourselves that it is their right to do so.

There may be good reasons why it is difficult for them to decide something: what to order in a restaurant, what career to pursue, or even what to wear.

'Ditherers' may be people who fear making a mistake. They may have grown up learning to do what other people want rather than risk causing upset by not choosing 'correctly'. They may agonise that, if they make the 'wrong' choice, they will 'miss out' and/or upset others.

We can support very young children in learning to choose by limiting their choices; e.g. 'Would you like to wear the red socks or the blue socks?' rather than 'What colour socks do you want to wear?"

We can support older children by helping them see the possible consequences of their choices; e.g. subject choice in school.

We can help adults who agonise about making decisions to verbalise what makes choosing so difficult for them. We can ask what they would say to someone in a similar situation.

We can remind them that, regardless of what they choose, we respect their right to make their own choices.

I feel … because I (think) … but I choose to:

Enjoy taking care of myself

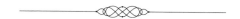

Taking care of ourselves might seem selfish.

It might seem too much hassle.

Taking care of others can make us feel good, kind and valued. Why does this not also apply to taking care of ourselves?

What would the world be like if we all deliberately valued taking care of ourselves and felt good about doing so?

I feel … because I (think) … but I choose to:

Remember that I was once three years old

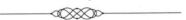

This Choose Well Statement supports me in different ways at different times.

Three-year-old children have wonderful possibilities.

They generally do not hide their feelings.

If they are happy, they laugh, and if they are sad, they cry.

They instinctively know how to play and tend not to worry about world politics, the weather, or if they have unintentionally upset someone.

I admire three-year-old children so much and when, at odd moments, I remember that I was once that age too, I smile.

I feel … because I (think) … but I choose to:

Allow myself to feel pain

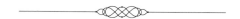

Have you been hurt recently?

You may have felt pain due to injury.

You may also have felt the pain of rejection or loss.

We often instinctively cover up and bury feelings of emotional pain.

We try to quickly pick ourselves up and 'pull ourselves together'.

Emotional pain hurts and we can fear that acknowledging this is to draw unwelcome attention to our pain or somehow make it even worse.

Choosing to allow ourselves to feel pain is one of the best things we can do for ourselves.

Once we become good at doing this, when we feel pain, we can allow ourselves to feel it, and then focus on what action we can take to help ourselves feel better.

I feel … because I (think) … but I choose to:

Act in a helpful way

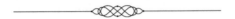

It is so easy to slip into 'unhelpful' habits in order to feel better.

For some of us, an unhelpful habit might be overindulging in unhealthy junk food.

It might be drinking alcohol excessively.

It might be avoiding or withdrawing from the challenges of life.

Choosing to act in a helpful way is not necessarily the easiest or the most enjoyable thing to do. It might involve doing the opposite of what we habitually and instinctively usually do.

This might be eating healthily, exercising when we would prefer to rest – or even resting when we would prefer to exercise!

One of life's important lessons is to figure out what exactly 'acting in a helpful way' means for us – and then choosing to do it.

I feel … because I (think) … but I choose to:

Allow myself to feel joyful

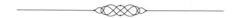

Have you noticed how sometimes it seems easier to feel upset, worried, hurt, sad, down, or even angry, than it is to feel happy, calm or joyful?

Why is this?

There are times in all our lives when we will feel burdened, hurt and heartbroken. We may not trust the moments we feel lighter, expecting them not to last and anticipating feeling even worse as a result.

It can be difficult, too, to feel joyful when others are struggling. We want them to know that we are there for them and it may seem wrong to enjoy feeling good when things are so hard for them.

It can be hard to allow ourselves to feel joyful, so let's start practising.

I feel … because I (think) … but I choose to:

Remember that 'A ship in harbour is safe, but that is not what ships are built for'

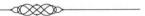

This quotation by John A. Shedd is one of my favourites and I find it helpful in gently nudging myself forward when I prefer to stay well within my comfort zone.

I also find the quotation helpful in encouraging people of all ages to rest in their harbour for a little while if they wish, but then to set off into the ocean of life knowing that they have the resources to cope with whatever happens on their voyage.

I feel … because I (think) … but I choose to:

Remember that 'Above the clouds, the sun is shining'

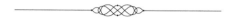

My favourite moment, when I am lucky enough to fly, is when the aeroplane breaks through the clouds into beautiful sunshine and blue skies.

When I stand on the ground on a wet, dull day, I enjoy looking at the clouds and reminding myself that the sun is up there, still shining, even if I cannot see it.

Knowing that 'above the clouds, the sun is shining' brings me particular comfort during life's difficult times.

I feel … because I (think) … but I choose to:

Celebrate my achievements

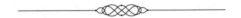

I sometimes ask people I work with to boast about themselves.

Typically, they look at me with surprise.

What do I mean, boast?

Yet they rarely hesitate as they tell me about all they have done wrong.

Why is it so hard for us to enjoy and even celebrate our achievements?

Apparently, the happiness that people who play sports feel when they win a particular match or tournament is fleeting.

The pain, upset, disappointment or even shame they feel when they lose can last longer.

What would it be like if we could stop, for even a few moments, to celebrate our achievements?

I feel … because I (think) … but I choose to:

Say 'Yes' to life

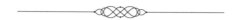

Although he died in 1997, Viktor Frankl's book *Yes to Life: In Spite of Everything* was published in English for the first time in 2020. His focus on the power we each have to choose to say yes to life, despite the challenges we encounter, is as relevant now as it was during the aftermath of the Holocaust.

Saying yes to life means that we acknowledge our feelings, regardless of how painful they may be.

Saying yes to life means that we become aware of and challenge our own thoughts and beliefs.

Saying yes to life means that we ask for, receive, accept and use support.

We live in a world of injustice, war, inequality and sickness. We also live in a world inhabited by resilient, courageous people who have each chosen to say yes to life and, just like Viktor Frankl, to make their lives count.

I feel … because I (think) … but I choose to:

Remind myself that challenges can strengthen me

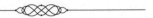

Every one of us faces challenges in life.

The German philosopher Friedrich Nietzsche said, 'What does not kill me makes me stronger.'

I am not too sure about this – I think it depends on how we choose to look at it.

People who have coped with horrendous difficulties have told me that they are stronger as a result.

Now when I find myself in a really challenging situation, I deliberately choose to remind myself that it can make me stronger.

I feel … because I (think) … but I choose to:

Welcome slips as learning opportunities

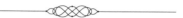

Sometimes people tell me that they thought they were doing well until they did something to let themselves down. The shame they feel is visible.

I ask them to think of mood as being on a scale from 0 to 10 (10 being high and 0 being low) and where they would position themselves on it. Most people opt for 6 or higher, with many choosing 9 or 10. I explain that while it is wonderful for us to have moments when life is at 9 or 10, we cannot stay there.

Often when I start to work with someone, their mood might be very low, and they might feel hopeless about life ever getting better. If they do something helpful such as deliberately planning and then doing one thing every day to give them pleasure (not alcohol-related and not necessarily costing money), their mood can lift.

As they begin to feel better, they may think, 'This is great!' but this can often be followed by a nasty inner voice telling them that the improvements will not last.

When something difficult happens, as it inevitably will, it can be accompanied by more nasty thoughts such as 'I told you it wouldn't work – you're useless and a complete failure.'

At those moments when we 'slip', it is vital to remember that we have a choice. We can choose to see our slips as failures.

Or we can deliberately choose to see them as learning opportunities.

This may be difficult but, if we can truly learn from them, these slips can provide the best learning opportunities we will ever have.

I feel ... because I (think) ... but I choose to:

Enjoy treating my body with respect

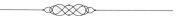

If we stand back from the marketing that constantly bombards us and ask, 'What are they telling me?', the answer is often that we are just not good enough.

To be better, we are told, we need to buy whatever is being advertised.

No beauty product, exercise machine, type of food or 'self-help' book is going to help if we do not use them wisely and correctly.

Choosing to treat our bodies with respect is a free choice.

It does not need to cost money and just think of the benefits in terms of health, well-being and self-respect.

The next time you notice yourself faced with a selection of sugary treats, considering whether to have another drink, or to buy a new beauty product, try saying to yourself, very clearly, 'I choose to enjoy treating my body with respect' – and see what happens.

I feel … because I (think) … but I choose to:

Develop good eating patterns

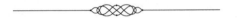

I like the word 'develop'. It inspires hope. Choosing to develop good eating patterns is powerful. If you arrive at an airport, your job is to get on the correct flight. It is not to fly the plane. The same goes for getting a taxi, or getting on a train. We know that someone else is employed to bring us where we want to go.

When we have thoughts such as 'I have to eat better', 'I should eat better', 'I can't eat better' or 'I must try to eat better', we are embarking on the journey of beating ourselves up because we think we are 'not good enough'.

When we have the thought, 'I choose to develop good eating patterns', we automatically focus on what that means. Good eating patterns may vary for each of us. It may mean sitting down to have a meal, away from the distractions of phone or television. It may mean that we eat smaller portions and stop eating when we are full. It may mean that we eat healthier.

Developing good eating patterns is more likely to happen when we deliberately choose to do so.

I feel … because I (think) … but I choose to:

Keep learning

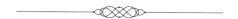

My friend Séan was midway through doing his PhD when he died. He was eighty-two and a lifelong learner.

I want to keep learning. There is a vast amount of evidence to prove that learning something new helps our brains as well as our sense of well-being.

Learning anything new means that we go through moments we enjoy and moments we find challenging. As we continue to learn, the basics become easier.

It then becomes easier to keep learning.

I feel … because I (think) … but I choose to:

Keep going

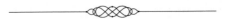

Have you ever had moments when you feel that you have just had enough? When you just want to stop rather than keep going? I have always liked the line from a poem I first read as a teenager, 'Don't Quit', by the American poet Edgar Guest:

'Rest if you must, but don't you quit.'

I think it is natural to have those moments when we feel overwhelmed, when it seems easier to stop rather than to keep going.

As the poem ends:

> Success is failure turned inside out,
> The silver tint of the clouds of doubt,
> And you never can tell how close you are.
> It may be near when it seems afar;
> So stick to the fight when you're hardest hit.
> It's when things seem worst that you must not quit.

So, choose to keep going!

I feel … because I (think) … but I choose to:

Gently pick myself up

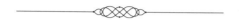

Have you ever noticed a young child running, falling, and waiting to be picked up?

A hug generally follows as the adult quickly checks that the child has suffered no serious harm.

There are times when I would so love someone to pick me up when I physically fall, or when I fall short of meeting an important goal.

Now I tend to give myself a few moments to acknowledge how I feel, link it to what I am thinking, and deliberately choose to gently pick myself up – and carry on as best I can.

I feel … because I (think) … but I choose to:

Stand and stare

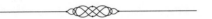

Another favourite poem of mine is 'Leisure' by the Welsh poet W.H. Davies. I particularly like the line:

> 'What is this life if, full of care, we have no time to stand and stare.'

The poem ends with the words,

> 'A poor life this if, full of care, we have no time to stand and stare.'

It is too easy to make a habit of rushing. Recently, I deliberately stopped in the middle of a beautiful forest, stood, and stared.

I heard the birds. I saw the buds on the trees. I felt the gentle breeze.

In gratitude for having stopped, I experienced a sense of peace and wonder that had just been there, waiting for me to stand and stare.

I feel ... because I (think) ... but I choose to:

Practise trust

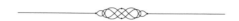

Some things take practice. Trusting can be one of those things.

'To be or not to be, that is the question' is a famous line from Shakespeare's play Hamlet.

A question many people might ask is whether to trust or not to trust.

Getting my car serviced is always done on trust. I have no idea what lies beneath the bonnet, and I trust whatever the mechanic tells me. I know that other people do not trust mechanics as easily as I do, but they may be more trusting in other situations.

When I was eleven years old, I learned to bake sponge cakes. My early attempts were completely ruined by my lack of trust in the oven doing its job without me opening the door every few minutes to check.

Sometimes it takes practice to trust!

I feel … because I (think) … but I choose to:

Get rid of the stuff I don't need

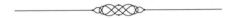

I was ten minutes into reading a new book before I realised it was the third book on 'decluttering' that I had bought in recent months.

My dilemma is that I have so many books I wonder whether I will ever have time to read them all.

Maybe I should get rid of them if I don't need them?

But what if I need them in the future?

How can I choose to get rid of what I don't need when I don't know whether I might need it again?

One of the authors of the decluttering books was very clear about this. Hoarding stuff that we think we might need someday takes up space. Getting rid of this stuff frees us up to do something else with the space and, if we do need these items in the future, we can buy them or, in the case of books, borrow them from the library.

I recently gave a bag of craft materials to someone who told me that they would use them in the next few weeks, rather than waiting for the day I might suddenly decide to use them myself. I am choosing not to get rid of many of my books, however, because I am not yet sure that I will never need them!

I feel … because I (think) … but I choose to:

Share

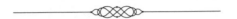

I sometimes feel sorry for little children when they get a treat and, just as they are about to tear it open, they are told to share it!

Have you ever seen the silent plea in the eyes of a child not to take the sweet or piece of chocolate that he is reluctantly offering you?

Yes, it is important that we all learn to share but sometimes it is hard to do so. Harder than we might expect!

Sharing does not have to mean that we end up with less of whatever it is we are sharing. Sharing, if done properly and with a good spirit, can mean that we gain rather than lose.

I am deeply grateful to people who share their expertise and time with me.

This includes the kind stranger who stopped when I was stranded on a motorway, discovering that 'knowing in theory' how to change a tyre did not help me actually change one.

Choosing to do something is not enough if we do not have the necessary skills or strength.

The consequences of choosing to share the skills we have with others tend to last much longer than the sweets we reluctantly shared when we were children.

I feel … because I (think) … but I choose to:

Develop self-control

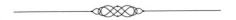

Picture yourself in a restaurant with friends. You're hungry and you know exactly what you want to order. The waiter respectfully waits for one of your friends to stop dithering over the menu. Do you feel frustrated? If so, what do you do? The polite and respectful reaction is for us to manage our own frustration in a way that does not involve snapping at someone to hurry up and order.

Waiting for someone to do something can be frustrating.

American psychologist Walter Mischel's book *The Marshmallow Test: Understanding self-control and how to master it* describes his famous 1960s experiment, the marshmallow test, when pre-school children sat on their own for twenty minutes in a room containing only a chair, a table and a treat they had chosen, such as a marshmallow. Each child was told that they could eat the treat whenever they wanted or wait for the adult to come back and then have two treats. Some children ate their treat moments after the researcher had left the room rather than wait to receive two treats instead.

Mischel describes how some children successfully resisted the temptation to eat their treat before the researcher returned by distracting themselves. Amazingly, children who exercised self-control at four years of age were found, years later, to be more successful in their studies, careers and relationships than children who immediately ate the treat.

Regardless of how difficult it is to resist temptation, we can all develop self-control.

I feel ... because I (think) ... but I choose to:

Allow others to experience the consequences of their choices

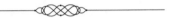

Perhaps one of the reasons we may rush in to decide for someone else is that we do not want them to experience upset or discomfort if they make what we consider to be the 'wrong' choice.

There is a Zen Buddhist story about a farmer who was philosophical when his horse ran away. It returned with two wild horses. His son broke one of his legs trying to tame them. War broke out. As a result of his injury, the boy was not chosen to fight.

The key point of this story is that we cannot know the consequence of any choice, and whether we will consider it to have been a 'good' or 'bad' choice, until the choice is made.

Susan Jeffers in her book *Feel the Fear and Do It Anyway* makes the interesting point that there are no 'good' or 'bad' decisions. She developed the 'No Lose' approach, which focuses on how to make our choices work for us.

One of my favourite films, *Heaven Can Wait*, illustrates this. A novice guardian angel rescues a man from the horrendous death he expects him to undergo in a motorcycle accident, not realising that the man would have survived if left to his own devices. I won't spoil the story, but it is an excellent portrayal of how 'rescuing' others from their choices can backfire.

Too often we try to 'rescue' others from what we believe will be a difficult consequence because doing this makes us feel better. However, this might not be the best action for them – or for us.

I feel … because I (think) … but I choose to:

Allow other people to learn what they choose to learn

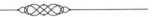

Teachers teach.

They cannot dictate or control what their students learn.

Neither can we.

Sometimes what we think is important for others to learn is wrong.

We might not know this.

They might not know this.

Choosing to allow others to learn whatever it is that they choose to learn means curbing our impulse to rescue, to control, to manage, and even to teach.

I feel ... because I (think) ... but I choose to:

Make my life count

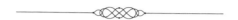

We have a wide range of choices in our lives.

The one that has become increasingly important to me is to make my life count.

What does 'making my life count' mean to you?

Your answer will depend on many things, such as your values, interests, abilities and life circumstances.

For me, the answer is summed up in the following lines, which are credited to the Quaker missionary Stephen Grellet (although they are sometimes attributed to others):

> I expect to pass through this world but once.
> Any good, therefore, that I can do
> or any kindness I can show to any fellow creature,
>
> let me do it now.
> Let me not defer or neglect it
> for I shall not pass this way again.

I feel … because I (think) … but I choose to:

Cherish the people I love

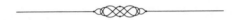

Many of us have become quite good at telling the people we love that we love them.

But do we cherish them as well as tell them that we love them?

You might say that part of loving someone is to cherish them.

I agree.

But it can be too easy to take the people we love for granted. Telling them that we love them can become an automatic response that might seem meaningless.

Cherishing them is different. It requires us to actively demonstrate our love.

It becomes easier to cherish the people we love when we remind ourselves to choose to do so.

I feel … because I (think) … but I choose to:

Give others space

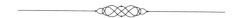

Teenagers are known for their desire for personal space.

But people of any age can crave space.

Space to feel exactly however they feel, without blocking or hiding their emotions.

Space to develop their creativity and personal interests.

Space in which they can see themselves as unique from everyone else.

Space to learn whatever they need to learn.

Space to enjoy.

What we see as 'enough space' might seem smothering and isolating to someone else.

Choosing to give others space will lead to us learning more about what space to give and when to give it.

I feel … because I (think) … but I choose to:

Recognise and appreciate what others do well

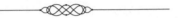

Sometimes, it can be hard to appreciate what others do well.

We filter their achievements through our 'I should have done better' lens.

While it might be easy to recognise what others do well, it can be difficult to genuinely appreciate their efforts.

We might not say that out loud.

We might dislike ourselves for our 'begrudgery'.

Instead of diving into self-blame and comparing ourselves unfavourably, how about we deliberately choose to recognise and appreciate what others do well?

It is even better if we tell them.

I feel ... because I (think) ... but I choose to:

Allow others space to slip, fall, and pick themselves up

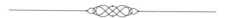

This fits with the 'curbing our impulse to rescue' theme.

It also requires us to allow others to have dignity and respect when they slip and fall.

It means that we support them in picking themselves up rather than ensuring that they stay down.

Let's generously choose to allow others the space to acknowledge their humanity in slipping and falling and their strength in picking themselves up.

I feel ... because I (think) ... but I choose to:

Celebrate other people's achievements

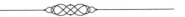

We live in a time in which we are bombarded with other people's achievements.

Social media grants us access to the lives of friends, acquaintances and complete strangers. Often, it is great to hear of their successes but, if we are not feeling good in ourselves, we can see others' achievements as proof of our own perceived inadequacies.

Choosing to recognise, appreciate and, even more, celebrate others' achievements, can be life-changing.

If we see other people's successes as somehow highlighting our own real or perceived inadequacies, we can better understand our reluctance to join in their celebrations.

Does everything, or nearly everything, have to be about us? Why can we not simply recognise someone else for who they are, and for what they are, without feeling smaller and more inadequate as a result?

I feel … because I (think) … but I choose to:

Allow others have their stories

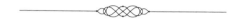

Has this happened to you?

You are listening to someone tell a story and someone else interrupts to correct them or to tell their own story instead.

As the title of Byron Katie's book *Who Would You Be Without Your Story?* reminds us, we each have a unique story. We can become very invested in these stories and come to see them as our identities.

What would it be like if we each allowed ourselves the space to come to terms with our stories?

Space to decide which of our stories we choose to bring with us as we grow older and which we choose to gently let go of?

How would it be if we deliberately chose to allow others to have their stories and give them opportunities to tell us about them?

Let's choose and see.

I feel ... because I (think) ... but I choose to:

Remember that others have the right to say 'No'

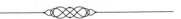

You may relate to this scenario. You have an idea. A good idea. Maybe even a great idea. It just depends on someone you know agreeing to do something. You feel excited and pleased. You ask the person for their help.

They say 'No'.

You feel annoyed and let down. Maybe they did not realise just how good your idea was. Maybe you did not explain it properly. So, you explain again what you want. This time you might be a little more forceful in attempting to be more persuasive. The person listens politely, then shakes their head while refusing, again, to do what you expected them to do.

You feel puzzled, initially. Then upset, frustrated and annoyed.

At this point you may start to plead. You may remind them of how obliging you always are when they ask you for a favour. You may cry. You may attempt to flatter or bribe them. You may even subtly threaten them.

The person continues to say 'No'.

You walk away feeling rejected, disappointed and annoyed. You wonder what you could have said to make them say 'Yes'. You tell yourself that you will remember this the next time they ask you for help.

How much easier would all this have been if you had deliberately chosen to remember that other people have the right to say 'No'?

I feel … because I (think) … but I choose to:

Respect the right of others to live their lives their way

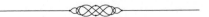

It is easy to choose to allow others to live their lives their way when it fits exactly with what we want. It can be totally different when they choose to live in a way that differs from our values, beliefs and expectations.

'But,' you might say, 'what if others choose to live in ways that have an adverse impact on my life, their own lives, or the lives of others?'

Article 6 of the Universal Declaration of Human Rights states that 'everyone has the right to recognition everywhere as a person before the law', while Article 7 states that 'All are equal before the law and are entitled without any discrimination to equal protection of the law.'

People are free to choose to live their lives as they wish. Before we cause them and ourselves distress by demanding that they change, it might be wise to reflect on whether they are breaking any law in our country – if they are not, our reactions might be our problem – not theirs.

I feel … because I (think) … but I choose to:
Set and maintain appropriate boundaries for any children I am responsible for

There are good reasons why children and young adolescents are not allowed to make certain decisions. This includes them not being mature enough to consider, or even see, possible consequences of their decisions. *Lord of the Flies* by William Golding illustrates this in a shocking and tragic way. While we are not going to abandon children to a desert island to live their lives however they want, it can be tempting to give in and allow them decide when they want to go to bed, what they want to eat, and even to make decisions, such as whether to go to school or not.

Setting and maintaining appropriate boundaries requires adults to know what is age-appropriate and fair. It also requires them to be independent of needing the child's approval. Support is available in the form of others who have been in the same situation as well as from parenting programmes such as Parents Plus and The Incredible Years, and from professionals such as GPs and psychologists.

Children of all ages need the adults who are responsible for them to be responsible in setting appropriate boundaries.

I feel ... because I (think) ... but I choose to:

Remember that others have the right to their opinions

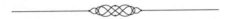

Conflict and unhappiness can result from insisting that others think the same way we do.

Reminding ourselves that others are entitled to their opinions, even if we do not agree with them, can be very freeing.

There are moments when we might look at other people with amazement, not understanding how they could possibly hold the opinions they do.

The book *Difficult Conversations: How to Discuss What Matters Most* by Douglas Stone, Bruce Patton and Sheila Heen offers an interesting approach to conflict resolution. Rather than doing our best to convince someone else that we are right, and they are wrong, it can be helpful to stand back like a neutral observer.

In most disputes, there is truth on both sides.

Reminding ourselves that others have the right to their opinions can help us negotiate common ground with respect and empathy.

I feel ... because I (think) ... but I choose to:

Treat others with respect

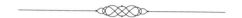

It is easy to treat people we regard highly with respect. It can be more challenging to show respect to people who live their lives in ways we may not approve of.

I remember reading a story about a man, Joe, who bought a daily newspaper from a shopkeeper who was always rude to him.

A friend who accompanied Joe into the shop one day was shocked to see just how appallingly the shopkeeper behaved. As they left, he asked Joe how he managed to continue to be polite and reasonable in the face of such rudeness.

Joe replied, 'Why would I allow someone else's bad behaviour to dictate how I behave?'

Some people respond to violence with violence. Others refuse to do so. They may stop for a moment to remind themselves that they have no idea why the other person is acting as they are. We do not need to condone unacceptable behaviour, but we owe it to ourselves and the world to deliberately choose to treat others with respect.

I feel … because I (think) … but I choose to:

Accept people's right not to love or accept me

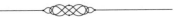

The theme of unrequited love dominates many poems, songs, books and films. Rejection seems cruel and can be very hard to take. The joys of 'young love' can turn to despair when one person decides that they no longer want to be in the relationship. The lyrics of the song 'The Girl from Ipanema' evoke what it is like to adore someone from afar while remaining invisible to them.

Unfortunately, some people do not accept someone's right not to love or accept them. As they harass and stalk the objects of their desire, they can be at best an irritation and at worst a threat to life.

Why do some people demand that others must love and accept them? Perhaps their demands lie in insecurity. Maybe they hand over entire responsibility for their well-being and happiness to someone else. When others love and accept them, they feel worthwhile – when they do not, they feel inadequate.

How much more relaxed would our world be if we each chose to accept people's right not to love or accept us?

I feel ... because I (think) ... but I choose to:

Be gentle with others who are going through a tough time

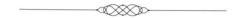

When one sports team is a player down in a match, the other team does its best to capitalise on their opponents' weakness.

Off the sports field, we can afford to be kinder.

When others struggle and are worn down by life, for whatever reason, we can deliberately choose to be gentle with them.

Of course, it is easier to be gentle with others when times are tough for them if we are good at being gentle with ourselves when times are tough for us.

I feel … because I (think) … but I choose to:

Allow others to be 'right'

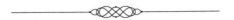

Sometimes, it is hard to allow others to be 'right'. Could this be because if they are right, we may be 'wrong'?

How would it be if each of us deliberately chose to allow others to be right?

They don't have to be wrong for us to feel good about ourselves. We don't have to be wrong for them to be right, either.

Let's move away from forcing others to be wrong so that we feel better about ourselves.

We might have different interpretations, different perceptions, and different beliefs.

Who am I to judge others as 'wrong'?

I choose to allow other people to be right and I look forward to seeing what happens as a result.

I feel … because I (think) … but I choose to:

Support others to do the best they can

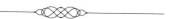

Not many people deliberately set out to offend or harm others.

We can take offence easily, regardless of whether it was meant or not.

We can criticise people for being too loud, too insensitive, too unkind, or too selfish.

We can complain because other people do not fit in with our views of how other people should be. Yes, there are times when people (including us) fall short of expectations.

There are times when people (including us) hurt others by their actions or inactions.

How about we stop the 'blame game' and look at what we can do better?

Let us each choose to support others in doing the best they can.

I feel … because I (think) … but I choose to:
Allow others to disagree with me

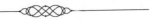

Learning to debate is an important life skill.

It assumes that others will disagree with us.

There is nothing wrong with this.

They might be 'right' in their views.

They might be 'wrong'.

They are entitled to have their views.

They are entitled to agree or disagree with my views.

Think of how freeing it would be if we could each choose to allow other people to disagree with us!

I feel … because I (think) … but I choose to:

Focus on other people's strengths

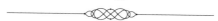

We have had the Ice Age and the Bronze Age – we may well now be living in the Hyper-Critical Age.

We know how destructive self-criticism is.

Focusing on what we consider to be 'weaknesses' in other people is destructive, too.

Every person on this planet has strengths.

There are times when we feel frustrated, upset or angry because we think that other people are just not good enough.

Choosing to change our perspective by deliberately focusing on their strengths can be very powerful.

It can help us see them in a different light. It can also encourage them to appreciate and maximise their own strengths.

Choosing to focus on other people's strengths can lead us from the Hyper-Critical Age to the Age of Kindness.

I feel … because I (think) … but I choose to:

Allow others to support me

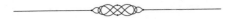

'Me do it' is a common phrase from a toddler who wants to do things his or her way.

As we grow up, we may prefer to do things ourselves and it can be difficult to accept support.

We might prefer to do things our way.

We might assume that others think 'needing help' means we are 'weak'.

We might not like doing things the way others want us to do them.

Being independent, being strong, and being capable are attributes that we tend to admire.

Supporting others can make us feel good.

Even the thought of needing support from others can make us feel bad.

During the COVID-19 pandemic, I came across Suzanne Jones's book *There is Nothing to Fix: Becoming Whole Through Radical Self-Acceptance*. It offered me support at a time when I did not know I needed it. Sue has developed a particular way of working with women (Trauma Informed Mind Body or TIMBo), which continues to transform my ability to manage my life's challenges.

Perhaps part of growing wiser as we grow older is realising that we cannot do everything ourselves. True strength, true independence and true humility lie in choosing to allow others to support us.

I feel ... because I (think) ... but I choose to:

Consider others

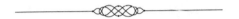

Would we have fewer wars, fewer arguments and fewer upsets if we each considered other people?

It is so easy to get locked into seeing the world from our own perspective.

Other people's successes or failures can be filtered through our own lens of how they impact us.

Let's choose to consider others.

If we do, if we really do, we will automatically treat them with kindness, with respect and, yes, with love.

We might even be better able to follow through on loving our neighbours as ourselves.

I feel ... because I (think) ... but I choose to:

Remember that my past is my past

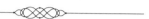

It can be tempting to look back on the past with nostalgia. We might think, 'Life was so much easier then.' Of course, we might also look back on the past with regret. We might think, 'Why did I do that?' and feel guilt and shame.

The pain of the past can cause pain in the present if we allow it to.

If we constantly compare our life now with how wonderful we consider it to have been in the past, we can rob ourselves of opportunities to make the most of our present.

The truth is that, regardless of whether we wish we were back in the past or whether we continue to be distressed by past experiences, our past is our past.

Choosing to remember that my past is my past and my present is my present can be a powerful and compassionate way of making the most of now.

I feel … because I (think) … but I choose to:

Do it willingly

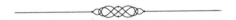

Many of the choices we make are influenced by people we have met and experiences we have had.

My mother often said, 'Do it willingly or don't do it at all' and 'Don't take the good out of it.'

I am reminded of her words when I realise that I have over-extended myself by offering to do something that 'seemed like a good idea at the time' but that turned out to be a lot more work than I had expected.

The habit of blaming myself kicks in automatically, followed by a few moments of grumpiness.

Then I hear my mother's voice and remember that I have choices.

I can choose not to do what I offered to do. I can do it while muttering and complaining silently to myself. Or I can choose to do it willingly.

I feel … because I (think) … but I choose to:

Be grateful

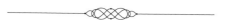

It is easy to be grateful when things are going well, although there can be a tendency to take good things for granted. Recognising that there is something to be grateful for can take practice.

There is wisdom in 'Count your blessings' but we can misinterpret that as 'Stop asking for more, you already have enough.'

A heartfelt thank you can mean so much. In the Irish language we often say, '*Míle buíochas*' – 'A thousand thanks' – as if one on its own could never be enough.

It can be difficult to be grateful for things that are difficult.

Yes, 'What does not kill us might make us stronger' but does that mean that we have to say 'Thank you' for it?

Choosing to be grateful for life's experiences changes our perspective. This can take time. Anyone who has experienced chronic illness, unemployment or homelessness will know that gratitude is an unlikely reaction in that context.

However, we may look back and see that we learned something that changed our lives for the better in a way that was not immediately clear at the time.

Choosing to be grateful opens us up to the possibility of experiencing gratitude at the right time, in the right way.

I feel … because I (think) … but I choose to:

Give myself every chance

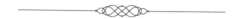

This book is about giving ourselves and others every chance – every chance to live our lives in a way that we can be proud of.

When I deliberately choose to give myself every chance, I find that I eat better, sleep better, exercise better and live better. Somehow, I am better able to resist temptation in whatever form it presents itself. Choosing to give myself every chance makes it easier to say 'No, thank you' to an extra slice of cake. It makes it easier to say 'Yes, please' to an invitation I might previously have rejected.

Choosing to give myself every chance means that I do what many of the Choose Well Statements highlight: I am kinder to myself. I am more understanding towards myself.

Choosing to give myself every chance puts me in a much better position to be there for others and to give them every chance, too.

I feel … because I (think) … but I choose to:

Remember that we have choices

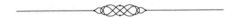

Sometimes, simply reminding ourselves that we have choices is enough to give ourselves every chance.

We don't have to put ourselves under pressure to make the right choice.

Remembering that we have choices reminds us that we can choose to breathe slowly.

Remembering that we have choices reminds us that we can ask for, receive and use support.

Remembering that we have choices reminds us that we are so much more than how we feel, what we think and what we do.

Remembering that we have choices reminds us that we are so much more than our experiences, fears and hopes.

Choosing to remember that we have choices is powerful.

Conclusion
I choose to choose well

Writing this book has been an interesting process. It has challenged me and it has surprised me. The original Choose Well Statement 'but I choose to cope' has been joined by many more. I hope that you have found some that resonate with you and that are helpful. I also hope that you choose to develop your own Choose Well Statements as you experience life's challenges in the future.

As I wrote this book, I was struck by how many of the Choose Well Statements focus on choosing to look after ourselves before looking after others. This makes sense. It is the idea of putting on your own oxygen mask before helping others put on theirs. It illustrates the idea that 'We cannot give what we do not have.' By choosing to take care of ourselves first, we are much better able to take care of others.

I teach what I need to learn. I always have done. As I teach people to acknowledge their feelings, to see them as making sense based on what is happening in their lives and/or on what they are thinking or doing, or to challenge their beliefs and focus specifically on helpful actions, I continue to learn. Working as a clinical psychologist does not mean that I am immune from stress, anxiety, disappointment, setbacks, frustration or grief. Doctors get sick. Plumbers can have burst pipes. Psychologists experience life challenges the same as everyone else.

Writing this book has highlighted for me how I have learned to better manage my particular life challenges in recent years. I use the ABC Coping Sentence on a daily basis and am constantly struck by how powerful it is. I love how it pulls key cognitive behavioural principles together in a simple and effective way.

This book contains ninety Choose Well Statements. The statements on their own are not enough. The real power comes from using them as part of the ABC Coping Sentence, 'I feel ... because I (think) ... but I choose to ...'

There will be moments when life's challenges seem overwhelming. These are the times to focus on one particular Choose Well Statement, which may be one of the most powerful of them all:

'I choose to choose well.'

May you choose well and may you enjoy choosing well.

Select Bibliography

SECONDARY SOURCES

Davies, W.H., *Songs of Joy and Others* (A.C. Fifield, 1911).

Dillard, Annie, *The Writing Life* (Harper Perennial, 2013).

Eger, Edith, *The Choice: Embrace the Possible* (Scribner, 2017).

—, *The Gift: 12 Lessons to Save Your Life* (Ebury Publishing, 2020).

Ehrmann, Max, *The Desiderate of Happiness* (Souvenir Press, 2017).

Frankl, Viktor, *Man's Search for Meaning* (Simon and Shuster, 1985).

—, *Yes to Life: In Spite of Everything* (Beacon Press, 2020).

Golding, William, *Lord of the Flies* (Faber and Faber, 1997).

Grellet, Stephen, *Memoirs of the life and gospel labours of Stephen Grellet* (E. Marsh Collection, 1862).

Hanratty, Malachy, *Discoveries in Prayer* (Columba Press, 2007).

Hayes, Claire, *Stress Relief for Teachers: The 'Coping Triangle'* (Routledge, 2006).

—, *How to Cope: The Welcoming Approach to Life's Challenges* (Gill, 2015; Bolinda, 2020).

—, *A Professional's Guide to Understanding Stress and Depression* (Institute of Chartered Accountants, 2016).

—, *Finding Hope in the Age of Anxiety* (Gill, 2017; Bolinda, 2020).

Jeffers, Susan, *Feel the Fear and Do It Anyway* (Ebury Publishing, 2014).

Jones, Suzanne, *There is Nothing to Fix: Becoming Whole Through Radical Self-Acceptance* (Suzanne E. Jones, 2019).

Katie, Byron, *Who Would You Be Without Your Story? Dialogues with Byron Katie* (Hay House, 2008).

King, David and Archard, Rhiannon, *A Hug for You* (Penguin UK, 2021).

Kübler-Ross, Elisabeth, with Kessler, David, *On Grief and Grieving: Finding the Meaning of Grief Through the Five Stages of Loss* (Simon and Shuster, 2014).

Mischel, Walter, *The Marshmallow Test: Understanding self-control and how to master it* (Transworld Publishers Ltd., 2014).

Nietzsche, Friedrich, *Twilight of the Idols* (Createspace Independent Publishers, 1889).

Ruiz, Don Miguel, *The Four Agreements: A Practical Guide to Personal Freedom* (Amber-Allen Publishing, 2018).

Shedd, John. A., *Salt from My Attic* (Mosher Press, 1928).

Stone, Douglas, Patton, Bruce and Heen, Sheila, *Difficult Conversations: How to Discuss What Matters Most* (Penguin, 2010).

Tatelbaum, Judy, *The Courage to Grieve* (Cedar Books, 1993).

SELECT ONLINE SOURCES

I Danced for the Angel of Death – The Dr. Edith Eva Eger Story: www.youtube.com/watch?v=WAguBQAFvto&t=10s

Suzanne Jones's website: https://www.timbocollective.org

Parents Plus: https://www.parentsplus.ie

The Incredible Years: https://incredibleyears.com

Acknowledgements

Whoever said that writing is a lonely experience has not yet met my family, friends, teachers, Síne Quinn, Fiona Dunne or the team in Beehive Books.

Within hours of Síne having received a draft of *Choose Well*, she responded with warmth and enthusiasm. With her talented 'Publisher hat' on, she ensured that the book received the very best editor (Fiona), the very best designer (Jeannie Swan) and the very best team (Lir Mac Cárthaigh, Jack Carey, Colette Dower, Leeann Gallagher, Kate O'Brien and all those in Beehive Books). While I am deeply grateful to Síne for her expertise and support as a gifted publisher, I am even more grateful to her for her kindness and encouragement.

Fiona added to my enjoyment in writing in unexpected ways. I was frequently struck by the care she took to ensure that my ideas were represented as well as they possibly could be. I began to think of her as the book's 'midwife' and now thank and celebrate her as the very best midwife (editor) this book could have had.

Sometimes the sign of a true craftsperson is when their work is almost invisible. This is true of the team in Beehive Books: each member of the team quietly and skilfully contributed to produce the beautiful book you now hold. I love what they have done and hope that you will, too.

Special thanks to Dr Ursula Bates, Patricia Scanlon and Dr Declan Lyons for endorsing this book. You may think that because they are kind, encouraging and absolutely lovely people, they would say nice things about this book, wouldn't they? That could well be true but they are each leaders in their fields and their recognition of the power of the 'ABC Coping Sentence' means more than I can say.

My teachers are too many to name but there are two I choose to include here, hoping that the rest will not mind. The first is Professor Mark Morgan, a lifelong mentor and friend. The second is 'George', who represents the people I am privileged to work with. Thank you.

Míle buíochas (one thousand thanks) are not enough to express my gratitude to my family and friends. You know who you are. You know how important you are in my life. You are there to celebrate lovely occasions (such as book launches) and, more importantly, you are there when times are tough.

Choose Well: The ABC Coping Sentence is my gift to each of you, *le míle, míle buíochas agus grá mór*.